Personal development f disability workers

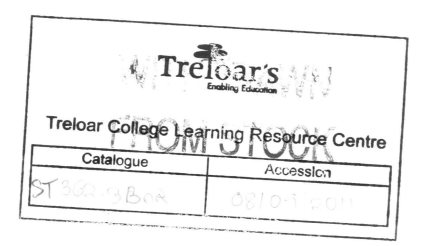

Series Editor: Lesley Barcham

Mandatory unit and Common Induction Standards titles

Communicating effectively with people with a learning disability
ISBN 978 0 85725 510 5

Personal development for learning disability workers ISBN 978 0 85725 609 6

Equality and inclusion for learning disability workers ISBN 978 0 85725 514 3

Duty of care for learning disability workers ISBN 978 0 85725 613 3

Principles of safeguarding and protection for learning disability workers
ISBN 978 0 85725 506 8

Person centred approaches when supporting people with a learning
disability ISBN 978 0 85725 625 6

Personal development for learning disability workers

Lesley Barcham

Supporting the level 2 and 3 Diplomas in
Health and Social Care (learning disability pathway)
and the Common Induction Standards

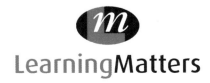
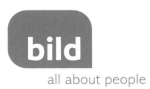

Acknowledgements

Photographs from www.crocodilehouse.co.uk and www.careimages.com. Our thanks to James Cooper, Autism Plus and Choices Housing for their help.

First published in 2011 jointly by Learning Matters Ltd and the British Institute of Learning Disabilities

British Library Cataloguing in Publication Data
A CIP record for this book is available from the British Library

ISBN: 978 0 85725 609 6

This book is also available in the following ebook formats:

Adobe ebook ISBN: 978 0 85725 611 9
EPUB ebook ISBN: 978 0 85725 610 2
Kindle ebook ISBN: 978 0 85725 612 6

Cover design by Pentacor
Text design by Pentacor
Project Management by Deer Park Productions, Tavistock
Typeset by Pantek Arts Ltd, Maidstone
Printed and bound in Great Britain by Ashford Colour Press Ltd, Gosport, Hants

Learning Matters Ltd
20 Cathedral Yard
Exeter
EX1 1HB
Tel: 01392 215560
E-mail: info@learningmatters.co.uk
www.learningmatters.co.uk

BILD
Campion House
Green Street
Kidderminster
Worcestershire
DY10 1JL
Tel: 01562 723010
E-mail: enquiries@bild.org.uk
www.bild.org.uk

Contents

> **This book covers:**
>
> - Common Induction Standards – Standard 2 – Personal development
> - Level 2 and Level 3 diploma units SHC 22 – Introduction to personal development in health and social care and children's and young people's settings and SHC 32 – Engage in personal development in health and social care and children's and young people's settings

About the author and the people who contributed to this book

Tina and James Cooper

James lives in his own bungalow in the Midlands and leads a full life in the community and with his family. He receives 24 hour support from a day service, a local care provider and his family. James loves swimming, music, going out to eat, watching football and motor racing. His mother Tina was James' main carer when he lived at home until three years ago. Tina and the rest of the family supported James to get his own home and arrange his support using a personal budget. Tina has supported other people with learning disabilities and their family carers to get a good life through self-directed support. Tina is a director of Time 4 People, an organisation that provides training, consultancy, presentations and information on all aspects of personalisation. For more information go to www.time4people.org.uk

Lesley Barcham

Lesley's career has been about learning. She trained as a teacher of deaf children in the 1970s and started out as a hearing therapist and then teacher of secondary aged deaf children. She has also worked in residential child care, teaching children with learning disabilities and adults with a learning disability in a further education college. Lesley gained a PhD from the Open University in the 1990s for her research into the development of education for disabled children in Southern Africa. Lesley has worked for BILD for 14 years on a variety of learning materials and programmes. From 2009 to 2011 she was seconded part time to the Valuing People Team as workforce adviser.

Introduction

Who is this book for?

Personal Development for Learning Disability Workers is for you if you:

- have a new job working with people with learning disabilities with a support provider or as a personal assistant;

- are a more experienced worker who is studying for a qualification for your own professional development or is seeking more information to improve your practice;

- are a volunteer supporting people with a learning disability;

- are a manager in a service supporting people with a learning disability and you have training or supervisory responsibility for the induction of new workers and the continuous professional development of more experienced staff;

- if you are a direct payment or personal budget user and are planning the induction or training for your personal assistant.

Links to qualifications and the Common Induction Standards

This book gives you all the information you need to complete both the Common Induction Standard on personal development, and the units *Introduction to personal development in health and social care and children's and young people's settings* (SHC 22) and *Engage in personal development in health and social care and children's and young people's settings* (SHC 32) from the level 2 and level 3 diplomas in health and social care. You may use the learning from this unit:

- to help you complete the Common Induction Standards;

- to work towards a full qualification, e.g. the level 2 or level 3 diploma in health and social care;

- as learning for the unit on personal development for your professional development.

This unit is one of the mandatory units that everyone doing the full level 2 and level 3 diploma must study. Although anyone studying for the qualifications will find the book useful, it is particularly helpful for people who support a person with a learning disability. The messages and stories used in this book are from people with a learning disability, family carers and people working with them.

Links to assessment

If you are studying for this unit and want to gain accreditation towards a qualification, first of all you will need to make sure that you are registered with an awarding organisation that offers the qualification. Then you will need to provide a portfolio of evidence for assessment. The person responsible for training within your organisation will advise you about registering with an awarding organisation and give you information about the type of evidence you will need to provide for assessment. You can also get additional information from BILD. For more information about qualifications and assessment go to the BILD website: www.bild.org.uk/qualifications

How this book is organised

Generally each chapter covers one learning outcome from the qualification unit, and one of the Common Induction Standards. The learning outcomes covered are clearly highlighted at the beginning of each chapter. Each chapter starts with a story from a person with a learning disability or family carer or worker. This introduces the topic and is intended to help you think about the topic from their point of view. Each chapter contains the following.

 Thinking points – to help you reflect on your practice.

Stories – examples of good support from people with learning disabilities and family carers.

 Activities – for you to use to help you to think about your work with people with learning disabilities.

Key points – a summary of the main messages in that chapter.

References and where to go for more information – useful references to help further study.

At the end of the book there is:

a glossary – explaining specialist language in plain English.

an index – to help you look up a particular topic easily;

Study skills

Studying for a qualification can be very rewarding. However, it can be daunting if you have not studied for a long time, or are wondering how to fit your studies into an already busy life. The BILD website contains lots of advice to help you to study successfully, including information about effective reading, taking notes, organising your time, using the internet for research. For further information, go to www.bild.org.uk/qualifications

Chapter 1

Competence in your work role with people with learning disabilities

During my first few days working with Adam and Eddie I was really all at sea. I felt overwhelmed by what I had to do, it was so different from shop work. Then after a week or so I got the hang of what Adam and Eddie wanted and needed me to do with them, but I had no idea if I was doing a good job to the right standard. Then my manager Kelly talked to me about the Code of Practice for social care workers and about the need to uphold people's rights under the Human Rights Act. It all started to make more sense then. Providing good support to Adam and Eddie was my first responsibility but there were also other external, bigger standards I needed to keep to as well.

Jenny – domiciliary care worker

Introduction

When you begin a new job or start work as a volunteer there is always so much to learn and find out. When you start work with people with learning disabilities it is essential that you focus on getting to know the people you support. A good understanding of your work role and the national standards you need to comply with will also help you see how the day-to-day support you provide fits into a bigger picture.

A growing number of workers are supporting people with learning disabilities who receive money for their support through a personal budget or direct payments. People can then, if they choose, directly employ their own workers as personal assistants or employ personal assistants through care support agencies. Personal assistants generally only support one person. They may be part of a small team of people providing individual support, so their situation is different from workers in more long-established organisations such as residential or day services.

Although there are lots of different roles supporting people with a learning disability and lots of different work settings, in any work role it is important to know from day one about your duties and responsibilities and the standards you need to work to.

Learning outcomes

This chapter looks at:

- understanding the main duties and responsibilities of your own work role;
- knowing about the standards and codes of practice that relate to your work role.

This chapter covers:

Common Induction Standards – Standard 2 – Personal development: Learning Outcomes 1.1 and 1.2

Level 2 SHC 22 – Introduction to personal development: Learning Outcome 1, assessment criteria 1.1 and 1.2

Level 3 SHC 32 – Engage in personal development: Learning Outcomes 1.1 and 1.2

Your main duties and responsibilities

Your duties and responsibilities, as a worker supporting a person with a learning disability, are summed up in your job title and then explained in more detail in your job description.

Your job title

Some job titles describe the job really clearly. For example, shop assistant, vet, gardener and social worker are familiar job titles and we know a bit about what they involve. But other job titles are not specific enough to tell you what the work is, let alone what day-to-day tasks are involved.

In your job supporting people with a learning disability your job title tells you and others about the work you do. You may be any one of the following:

support worker   *home carer*   *personal assistant*

job coach   *care assistant*

These titles tell you something about the job, but not very much. Two people with the same job title may in fact do very similar work or their duties may be very different. It's then that your job description is helpful as it gives you much more information about your duties and responsibilities.

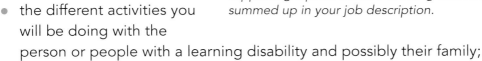

Thinking point

What is your job title? Does it describe what you do? When you tell your family and friends what your job title is, do they completely understand what you do every day?

Your job description

As a learning disability worker, you should have received a job description when you applied for your job. When you started in your current job your line manager should go through your job description with you in detail. A job description covers:

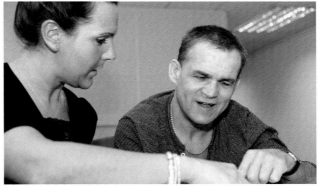

Your duties and responsibilities, as a worker supporting a person with a learning disability, are summed up in your job description.

- the different activities you will be doing with the person or people with a learning disability and possibly their family;

- your responsibilities;

- who you are accountable to.

Although job descriptions can vary from organisation to organisation, or from person to person, and some may still not be very detailed, your job description is an important document for you in your job as a learning disability worker.

If you are a volunteer you are unlikely to have a job description, but you may well have a written task or role description which should contain some or all of:

- your title;
- the purpose of your role;
- who you are responsible to;
- the activities or tasks you will be involved in.

The task description could also include additional information on the time and location of your volunteering and also any policies you need to follow, for example on confidentiality, health and safety. Many organisations now have a volunteer's code of conduct. If the organisation you volunteer with has one, make sure you have read it through and discussed it with the volunteer co-ordinator.

As well as looking at your role and responsibilities it's a good idea to look at the aims and values of your organisation. When you are clear what these are it can be easier to see how your day-to-day contribution helps your organisation work towards its goals.

An aim is a general statement of what an organisation hopes to achieve in its work with people with learning disabilities. Some organisations put their aims into a mission statement or vision statement. Find out if your organisation uses these terms. Values are statements about what an organisation considers to be important in its work with people with learning disabilities. They are the expression of the beliefs and opinions on which the organisation was founded and underpin the way that it operates. Values inform the aims of an organisation. For example, your organisation may have as one of its values that all people are individuals and everyone's unique qualities, ability and experience are valuable assets. This means that you should identify, celebrate and promote the skills, talents and understanding of each person you support in your daily work.

Every organisation has a set of aims and values. You should have been given information about them at your interview and talked about them during your induction. Have you really thought about what they mean, and how they help you do your job?

Thinking point

Look at the aims and values of the organisation you work for. How have you contributed to achieving them in your work with people with a learning disability over the last few days?

If you are working as a personal assistant employed by one person, you are unlikely to have information on the aims and objectives of an organisation, but what you might well have, if the person wants to share them with you, is a copy of all or part of their person centred plan or their support plan. These should direct you with your values and give important information about the person's aims in life. Your role is to support them in achieving them.

To know what your duties and responsibilities are in your job supporting a person with a learning disability, you need to look at:

- your job title;
- your job description;
- the aims and values of the organisation you work for;
- the person-centred plan or support plan of the person you support.

Standards for social care workers

As well as having duties and responsibilities to the people you support and the organisation that employs you, you also have wider responsibilities as one of over one million social care workers in the UK. These standards and responsibilities are set out in:

- the Code of Practice for social care workers;
- the Human Rights Act and other overarching laws;
- the requirements for the inspection and regulation organisations for health and social care services in your country;
- National Occupational Standards.

The Code of Practice

The Code of Practice for social care workers in England says that all workers must:

- protect the rights and promote the interests of service users and carers;
- strive to establish and maintain the trust and confidence of service users and carers;
- promote the independence of service users while protecting them as far as possible from danger or harm;
- respect the rights of service users while seeking to ensure that their behaviour does not harm themselves or other people.

The Code of Practice also states that as a social care worker, you must protect the rights and promote the interests of service users and carers. This includes:

- treating each person as an individual;
- respecting and, where appropriate, promoting the individual views and wishes of both service users and carers;
- supporting service users' rights to control their lives and make informed choices about the services they receive;
- respecting and maintaining the dignity and privacy of service users;
- promoting equal opportunities for service users and carers;
- respecting diversity and different cultures and values.

Thinking point

Look at just one of the points from the list above on protecting people's rights and respecting their views. Think about how you can demonstrate that you work in this way.

The social care councils for each of the four countries of the UK were set up by the government in 2001 to register and regulate all social care workers.

The General Social Care Council in England, the Care Council for Wales, The Northern Ireland Social Care Council and the Scottish Social Services Council all published Codes of Practice for Social Care Workers in 2002.

You should always work to the standards set out in the Code of Practice for the country you work in. They set out standards relating to professional conduct and practice that are required of all social care workers. You will find that many of these are similar to those from your own organisation, but the difference is that these are set at a national level and have been devised to ensure people who are supported, their families, carers and other members of the public know the standards of conduct they should expect from social care workers.

In relation to your accountability as a social care worker the Code of Practice says that you must:

> *6.1 Meet relevant standards of practice and work in a lawful, safe and effective way*
>
> *6.8 Undertake relevant training to maintain and improve your knowledge and skills and contributing to the learning and development of others*

This is why it is important for both new and experienced workers to know about the current standards and legislation and how they apply to their work. Regular updates are important so that you keep abreast of changes and developments.

National laws

In any job that you do there are laws and regulations that you need to know about and follow. Health and safety at work laws relate to all work settings. You need to know what the laws and regulations on health and safety at work mean to you in your workplace. So for example, what does the law say about moving and handling a box at work and what does it say about supporting a person to move from their bed to a wheelchair?

Then there are more specific laws and regulations that you need to know about that are about health and social care and supporting people with a learning disability. For example, there are laws on safeguarding children and vulnerable adults, mental capacity and confidentiality that will have a direct impact on your work.

A number of other books in this series look in detail at national laws and regulations relating to a particular topic, for example health and safety and safeguarding. This section focuses on the key laws that contribute to the overarching principles and standards in social care work.

The Human Rights Act 1998 came into force in the UK in October 2000, and brought most of the rights in the European Convention on Human Rights into our domestic law. The Human Rights Act ensures respect for human rights for everyone and of course this includes people with a learning disability.

The Act means that all public authorities and other bodies performing public functions in the UK (such as private companies providing health and social care support) must respect the rights contained in the Human Rights Act in everything that they do. If you work for a public authority such as a council, hospital or college then you are under a duty to respect the rights of the people with learning disabilities. Also if you work for a voluntary sector or private care provider that is providing public services such as social care, you too must work within the Act. Everyone is protected by the Human Rights Act – including people with learning disabilities, their family carers and the workers supporting them. The following rights are protected by the Act.

WHAT RIGHTS ARE PROTECTED BY THE HUMAN RIGHTS ACT?

- Right to life
- Freedom from torture, inhuman and degrading treatment
- Freedom from slavery and forced labour
- Right to liberty and security
- Right to a fair trial
- No punishment without law
- Right to respect for private and family life
- Freedom of thought, conscience and religion
- Freedom of assembly and association
- Freedom of expression
- Right to marry and found a family
- Right not to be discriminated against in your employment of your other human rights
- Right to peaceful enjoyment of your possessions
- Right to free elections
- Right to education

Human rights abuses are going on every day in our communities suffered by people with learning difficulties and it is time something was done about it. This quote from Andrew Lee, a director of People First and a self-advocate with a learning disability, sums up many people's experience. People with a learning disability say that in their experience their rights are not upheld, particularly in relation to:

- the right to life;
- freedom from inhuman and degrading treatment;
- the right to liberty;
- the right to respect for private and family life, home and correspondence;
- the right not to be discriminated against.

Unfortunately we also know from a number of investigations into bad practice and abuse that people with a learning disability often have their human rights breached. A joint parliamentary report on human rights and people with a learning disability said that there are still real concerns about people with learning disabilities not being afforded the same human rights as everyone else. It also says it is vital that public services take a positive, proactive approach to protecting, respecting and fulfilling the human rights of people with learning disabilities.

Supporting and promoting the human rights of people with a learning disability as set out in the Human Rights Act is an essential part of being a learning disability worker. This means that you should take a human rights-based approach in all that you do. This includes:

- having as your starting point the view that all people have rights;
- treating everyone you meet in the course of your work with dignity and respect;
- not discriminating against anyone because of their age, gender, disability, religion, ethnicity or sexual orientation;

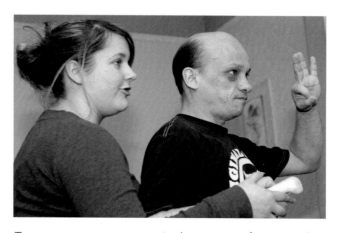

Treat everyone you meet in the course of your work with dignity and respect.

- using your knowledge of the rights protected by the Act to inform the way you work and also to enable the people with learning disabilities that you support to get their rights.

As well as knowing about the Human Rights Act, workers supporting people with a learning disability also need to be guided by the standards set out in the Equality Act.

> **The Equality Act 2010** brought together under one law all previous laws about discrimination in Britain (Northern Ireland is not covered by the Act). The Equality Act provides legal protection against discrimination under six equality strands: sex, race, disability, age, religion or belief and sexual orientation. The law protects people against direct and indirect discrimination, discrimination by association, harassment and victimisation. (For more information look at the *Equality and Inclusion for Learning Disability Workers* book in this series.)

Your employer needs to take these key national laws and the more specific legislation very seriously and make sure that they and their workers don't break the law. You will find that your employer has used the laws to help them write policies and procedures. New workers need to know about the policies and procedures of the organisation they work for and what they mean in their day-to-day work. During your induction you should find out about all the policies and procedures that relate to your day-to-day work with people with a learning disability. Keeping to the policies and procedures will mean that you are keeping to the standards set out in the Code of Practice and the national laws.

Registration and inspection standards

Many health and social care providers are inspected by an independent regulator. There are different regulators for the four countries of the UK. They are:

- the Care Quality Commission (CQC) for England;
- the Care and Social Services Inspectorate for Wales;
- the Social Work Inspection Agency in Scotland;
- the Regulatory Quality and Improvement Authority in Northern Ireland.

Depending on the country, the independent inspection agency will regulate hospitals, care homes, day care and organisations providing support in the person's own home. Inspections usually cover public, private and charity sector providers. The aims of inspection bodies are to make sure high quality care is provided for everyone.

Each inspection agency has its own standards and outcomes against which it checks people's experiences of services. For example, the CQC for England has as one of its essential standards of quality and safety that providers should respect and involve people who use services. This would mean that if you worked in a CQC inspected services, you and your work colleagues would need to provide information on how you promoted people's dignity and respect as well how people with a learning disability and family carers are involved in giving feedback on the organisation.

Activity

Find out from your manager whether the organisation you work for is inspected by an independent quality agency. If you work for a regulated and inspected service find out a bit more about the standards they use for inspection by going to the appropriate website.

Other standards for social care workers

As well as standards relating to inspection there are other standards for the social care worker that come from the sector skills councils for each country. For example, in 2008 Skills for Health and Skills for Care in England in their *Common Core Principles of Self Care* set out seven principles for workers supporting people with their health and social care.

Common core principles of self-care

- Ensure individuals are able to make informed choices to manage their self-care needs.
- Communicate effectively to enable individuals to assess their needs, and develop and gain confidence to self-care.
- Support and enable individuals to access appropriate information to manage their self-care needs.
- Support and enable individuals to develop skills in self-care.
- Support and enable individuals to use technology to support self-care.
- Advise individuals how to access support networks and participate in the planning, development and evaluation of services.
- Support and enable risk management and risk taking to maximise independence.

These principles underpin the Common Induction Standards and the new health and social care diploma so by reading this book and undertaking learning as a new worker you will find out how to put these principles into practice.

In addition, campaigns relating to providing good support for people who use health and social care services, such as the Department of Health's Dignity in Care campaign, set out very clear challenges for workers. Three of their ten challenges say workers should:

- support people with the same respect you would want for yourself or a member of your family;
- treat each person as an individual by offering a personalised service;
- enable people to maintain the maximum possible level of independence, choice and control.

For more information on how you can use the dignity challenge go to www. dignityincare.org.uk/DignityCareCampaign/

National Occupational Standards

In starting work as a learning disability worker and as you develop in your role you may find the national occupational standards useful in understanding the knowledge, skills and competencies needed to do a good job. National occupational standards (NOS) describe the skills, knowledge and understanding needed to undertake a particular task or job to a nationally recognised level of competence. You can download the NOS for adult social care from the Skills for Care website at www.skillsforcare.org.uk

You can use the NOS to:

- carry out a self-assessment of your current competences. This can help you think about the learning you need to do and any skills you will need to develop if you want to change jobs;
- plan your own personal development as the NOS give information on what you need to learn to gain a qualification or progress in your role.

As well as individual workers using National Occupational Standards to assess and plan their learning, employers can also use them to:

- describe the skills they need in their workforce;
- assess the skills already in the workforce;
- develop training and recruitment plans to fill any identified gaps and shortages;
- form the basis of job descriptions;
- set objectives in performance and appraisal;
- develop and evaluate training for both individuals and the organisation.

This information has come from the UK Standards organisation. You can find out more about NOS at www.ukstandards.org.uk.

You can see from this chapter that your own job duties and responsibilities are informed by national laws, the values and aims of the organisation you work for, and your responsibilities as a social care worker, as in the following diagram:

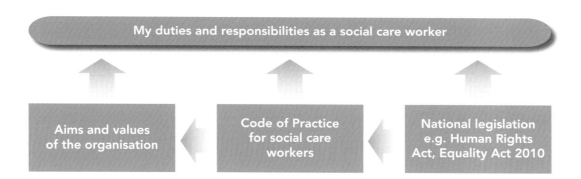

You will have been given information about your role and responsibilities at your interview and during your induction to your new job. However, you are bound to find yourself in situations in which you are unclear about the limits of your own responsibility, and you need help and advice from others.

Key points from this chapter

- As a worker supporting people with a learning disability there are a number of different standards that you should know about and be working to. Together they are summed up by these six points.

1. Protect and promote the person's human rights.

2. Promote the person's independence while working with them to ensure their safety.

3. Treat everyone with dignity and respect.

4. Promote choice and control for all the people you support.

5. Respect diversity.

6. Respect the person's confidentiality.

References and where to go for more information

References

BIHR (2008) *The Human Rights Act – Changing Lives,* second edition. London: BIHR

Fulton, R and Richardson, K (2011) *Equality and Inclusion for Learning Disability Workers.* Exeter: Learning Matters/BILD

Skills for Care and Skills for Health (2008) *Common Core Principles to Support Self Care.* Leeds: Skills for Care

Legislation, policies and reports

All UK legislation can be downloaded from www.legislation.gov.uk

Policies and reports for Northern Ireland, Scotland and Wales can be found at www.northernireland.gov.uk www.scotland.gov.uk and www.wales.gov.uk respectively. Policies and reports for England can be found on the website of the relevant government department.

Report of House of Lords and House of Commons Joint Committee on Human Rights (2008) *A Life Like Any Other? Human Rights of Adults with Learning Disabilities Seventh Report of Session 2007–08.*

Human Rights Act 1998

Equality Act 2010

Websites

British Institute of Human Rights www.bihr.org.uk

British Institute of Learning Disabilities www.bild.org.uk

Care and Social Services Inspectorate Wales (CSSIW) www.csiw.wales.gov.uk

Children's Workforce Development Council www.cwdc.org.uk

Equality and Human Rights Commission www.ehrc.org.uk

Skills for Care www.skillsforcare.org.uk

Skills for Care and Development www.skillsforcareanddevelopment.org.uk

Social Work Inspection Agency (Scotland) www.swia.gov.uk

The Social Care Councils (responsible for the regulation and registration of Social Workers and other Social Care Workers) are:

General Social Care Council (England) www.gscc.org.uk

Care Council for Wales www.ccwales.org.uk

Northern Ireland Social Care Council www.niscc.info

Scottish Social Services Council www.sssc.uk.com

Chapter 2
Being a reflective worker and evaluating your practice

I want the staff that support James to put themselves in his shoes and be truly person centred in all that they do. Although everything is written down in James's support plan and they have training from us, his family and their employer they still don't always get it right. Some of the best workers are the ones who ask questions and think about what has gone right and why sometimes things go wrong. As James's mum I am always thinking about his support, reflecting on things, looking for ways to do things differently, better. I want and expect the same from the managers of the organisation that support James and the support workers. Then James gets a good life and he stays safe, healthy and happy.

Tina Cooper, family carer, mother of James

Introduction

The people with learning disabilities you support and their families have a right to expect high quality care from you and the service you work for. You have a responsibility to always provide the best possible support that you can to a high standard. One important way to learn and improve what you do, whether you are a new worker or have worked in care for many years, is to be a reflective worker. In this chapter we look at reflective practice, why

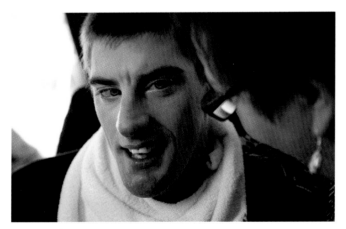

Tina and James.

it is important and how to demonstrate that you are a reflective worker. The chapter also looks at how you can assess your own knowledge and skills and why communication, literacy and numeracy skills are important when you are supporting a person with a learning disability.

Learning outcomes

This chapter looks at:

- how your values, attitudes and experiences affect the support you provide and can be a barrier to doing a good job;

- reflective practice: what it is and why is it important;

- demonstrating how you use reflective practice to improve the support you provide.

This chapter covers:

Common Induction Standards – Standard 2 Personal development: Learning Outcomes 1.3, 2.1 and 2.2

Level 2 SHC 22 – Introduction to personal development: Learning Outcomes 1–1.3 and 2

Level 3 SHC 32 – Engage in personal development: Learning Outcome 2

How your values, attitudes and experiences affect the support you provide

Thinking point

Look at these three newspaper headlines and be honest with yourself about what your reaction was to each story.

Man with learning difficulties 'tortured and forced off a viaduct to his death'

A man with severe learning difficulties was violently tortured for hours before being forced to take 70 painkillers and falling from a viaduct to his death, a court heard.

Daily Mail 13 June 2007
www.dailymail.co.uk/

Voice for a new age

The young, relatively unknown Scott Watkin, who has gone from supermarket shelf-stacker to learning disabilities co-director in the Department of Health, tells David Brindle that his advisory role on developing strong advocacy is anything but tokenistic.

The Guardian 20 May 2009
www.guardian.co.uk/

A hug for Prince of Wales, the prince of hearts

Prince William is hugged by Darren Pearty as he meets children at Eresby Special School in Lincolnshire.

Daily Mail 11 January 2010
www.dailymail.co.uk/

What were your immediate reactions to these headlines?

- It's terrible that people with learning disabilities are victims of hate crime.
- This is so unjust, what can I do about this?
- People should be in a safe place like a home so bad people can't hurt them.
- Children and adults with learning disabilities are all loving and like hugging people.
- People with disabilities should receive charity from rich and famous people.
- More people with learning disabilities should get jobs; they can be good workers.
- I don't think people can get work, they all need to be cared for.
- All people have the same human rights and should be treated with dignity and respect.

How you reacted to these stories gives you an indication about your current values and beliefs about people with a learning disability. It is important to be honest about what these are as they will influence how you behave when you support a person with a learning disability. For all of us our values and attitudes are a result of a complex mix of things that have come together to shape our current views.

Factors that influence our values and attitudes towards people with a learning disability

Your family, early years experiences and your friends – the values that you were taught as a child from your close family and school are important even in adult life. Also the ideas and views that you picked up as a young adult from friends and your current friends and acquaintances.

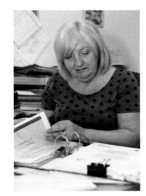

The communities you belong to – what do the people you spend your free time with think about people with disabilities and people with learning disabilities? If you have strongly held political or religious views, how are these affecting your views of people with a learning disability?

Your work situation – as a new learning disability worker you will be strongly influenced by the values and behaviour of your manager and co-workers as well as those of the family carers and friends of the people you support.

The wider cultural, social values and attitudes – how do the films and television programmes you watch show people with a learning disability? What about the newspapers and magazines that you read or the websites you visit?

A recent survey (2010) was carried out by a national charity Turning Point asking 1000 adults about their understanding of people with a learning disability. Here are some of the headlines from that poll.

1. A third of Britons think people with learning disabilities cannot live independently or do paid work.
2. Almost a quarter imagined they would be living in care homes.
3. Nearly one in ten (8 per cent) expected them to be cared for in a secure hospital out of town.

4. Nine out of ten thought they experienced discrimination, half (51 per cent) thought they were the most discriminated against group in society — coming above other groups often perceived to experience discrimination, including gay people (44 per cent), overweight people (43 per cent) and ethnic minorities (40 per cent).

5. A third thought mental illness was a learning disability.

So if when you start work with people with a learning disability some of your values and attitudes are similar to those of the people who answered the Turning Point survey, don't be too harsh on yourself. Rather take this as an opportunity to reflect on your current attitudes and use your reflection to think about the values and attitudes you will need to be a good learning disability worker. This is the start of being a reflective practitioner, an important aspect of providing good support.

How can I make sure that my values, attitudes and experiences are not a barrier to doing a good job?

Having the right attitude towards people with a learning disability is the most important thing when recruiting new support workers. Treating us with respect and listening to what we say is top of our list.

Andy, self-advocate involved in recruiting new staff

As you can see from this quote, treating the people you support with dignity and respect, listening carefully to what they are saying and acting on it are some of the most important attitudes that people with a learning disability tell us they want from the people who support them.

In Chapter 1 you can see that there are standards and laws that all social care workers need to keep to. You may find this difficult sometimes in your work. Here are a few of the possible conflicts you might experience.

1. You may find it much easier to work with one person but you really don't get on with someone else, so you spend less time with them.

2. You find it hard to respect the choices of the person you support – you think you know best. You think they are making unwise or dangerous choices.

3. You think the parents of a person you support are overprotective, therefore you don't listen to their ideas at all. You focus on what the person says they want.

If on reflection you think that maybe some of your values and attitudes are a barrier to providing good support there are number of practical steps you can take to address this. Instead of feeling bad, rather being honest about how you feel and finding a solution is a positive and brave thing to do. It will help you develop into a really good worker. Look at the three stories below and the steps the worker took to make sure their values weren't a barrier to providing good support.

Barriers to providing good support

Ginnie had never supported anyone from a Jewish background before. She didn't understand Simon's insistence that he always have kosher food when they are out, even when he was really hungry.

Ronan always had to go through his rituals and routines when they left his house to go to the day service. Jamie found it annoying and he got impatient and wanted to tell him to hurry up as they were often late.

Overcoming barriers to providing good support

To Ginnie, Simon's insistence that he eat certain food for religious reasons was difficult to understand. She was an atheist, loved her food and was concerned that Simon's behaviour might affect his diabetes and she would be to blame.

Ginnie talked to both Simon and his brother about what would be suitable snacks for him to have when he is out. Ginnie realised she couldn't discriminate against Simon on religious grounds and that she needed to find out more about Jewish religious practices.

Ronan has autistic spectrum condition and going through certain routines and rituals helps him manage difficult transitions such as leaving the house or changing activities. Jamie talked to his manager about his impatience and annoyance at his next supervision. Reflecting with his line manager he realised that although he knew a bit about autism he needed to understand more about what having autism meant for Ronan. He read Ronan's person-centred plan, watched a DVD about supporting people with autism and talked again to his manager. Once he knew Ronan better and about his autism he wasn't so impatient and he left more time for Ronan to do things at his pace.

Louise just didn't get on with Jane when she came to live in the residential home where she worked. Jane was quiet and sad as her dad had just died. She enjoyed doing things at home and didn't want to go out. The other two women in the home were much younger, more outgoing, liked lots of music and fun and the staff got on really well with them. Jane became more withdrawn after being at the home for two months.

Louise was irritated by Jane because she just didn't fit into the home and how things were run. The staff and the other two women had got a system that worked for them and it was all disturbed by Jane.

Jane's advocate challenged Louise and asked her if the staff in the home believed in person centred support because this wasn't Jane's experience. This really made Louise think and she realised that they were trying to make Jane fit into the services and they were not looking at her needs. Louise realised that what they were doing was not right. With Jane and her advocate she started to support Jane to develop her own person centred plan.

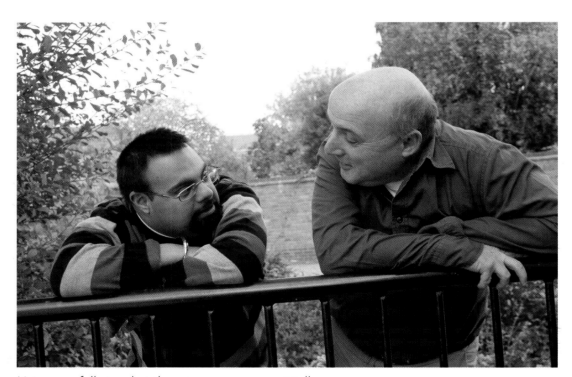

Listen carefully to what the person you support tells you.

If you think that your values and attitudes might be a barrier to providing good support you can:

- talk to your manager or an experienced work colleague;
- learn more about the person you are supporting, their strengths, dreams and needs;
- read the Code of Practice and other documents that set out the standards you need to work to;
- look at different ways to get the information or skills you need to be a better worker;
- listen carefully to any compliments or complaints and take action when it's needed.

What is reflective practice and why is it important?

I found Beth's noisy and agitated behaviour challenging to manage when we went to the swimming pool, it was so unlike her. After talking to her mum and thinking about what had changed recently, I realised it was just too busy and loud for Beth when we went during the school holidays. Earlier in the day or when it was quieter was much better.

Ruth, personal assistant

Working with other people is always complex. There is lots to consider and however hard we try we don't always get it right. Reflection is a way to learn from our past experiences, both good and bad, so that we can get better at what we do. Reflective practice is an organised way to think through, either on your own or with others, what has happened in your support of a person with a learning disability so that you can change what you do for the better. Reflective practice is practical learning directly from life, not from a book or a course; instead it is learning by taking a new, critical look at our own experiences.

Getting into the habit of being a reflective worker from your first days supporting people with a learning disability and then carrying it on throughout your career in social care will help you to continually learn and improve.

Think back to one thing that went really well in your support of a person with a learning disability in the last week. Now think about one thing that didn't go so well. Why do you think things happened as they did?

How can I use reflective practice to improve the support I provide to people with a learning disability and their families?

In everyday life we are always learning from our experiences. When something goes well we can use our knowledge of why it went well in similar situations. If something goes really badly we often go over and over it in our minds or in discussion with others, trying to work out why. Similarly in your day-to-day work, by developing a habit of regularly reflecting on what you do, you can improve how you support people.

Reflecting on a situation can be seen as a number of stages. We have illustrated this using Ruth's story above.

- **Stage 1 – Description – What happened?** Something different or out of the ordinary happens in your day-to-day support of a person with a learning disability.
  For Ruth, one day out of the blue Beth's behaviour changed when they went to the swimming pool.

- **Stage 2 – Feelings – What were you thinking and feeling?** Think through the event and remember how you felt.
  Ruth felt surprised and shocked that she wasn't able to cope well when Beth started shouting and then crying. She hadn't predicted this would happen and was unprepared.

- **Stage 3 – Evaluation – What was good and bad about the experience?** Remember both the positive and negative consequences of the event.
  Ruth felt bad because while she was looking after Beth she had got distressed in a situation that they had been in successfully together many times before. The good point from the incident for Ruth was that once she realised that the noise level and crowds in the pool were distressing Beth, she cut short the swimming and they went to a quiet cafe that Beth liked.

- **Stage 4 – Analysis – What sense can you make of the situation?** On reflection how do you explain what happened?

  Later Ruth spoke to Beth's mum about what happened. Her ideas together with her own recollection of when Beth had reacted in a similar situation helped Ruth realise that it was the noise level that had distressed Beth.

- **Stage 5 – Conclusion – What else could I have done?** How could you manage the situation differently?

  Ruth's conclusion was that loud crowded situations are too much for Beth and that if they go into such a situation again together she should try and divert her into a different, quieter activity before she gets too distressed.

- **Stage 6 – Action plan – If it arose again what would you do?** Should such an incident happen again what could you do differently?

  Ruth decided to talk to Beth about swimming at a quieter time of day, especially in the school holidays when the pool is very busy. In a similar noisy situation Ruth has agreed with both Beth and her mum that the best thing is to leave the situation and go somewhere quieter.

This six stage process is based on a well-known theory of learning and reflection developed by Graham Gibbs (1988). There are a number of other reflective models that you could use developed by, for example, Kolb. However, using the Gibbs model to start with will help you in developing your reflective skills.

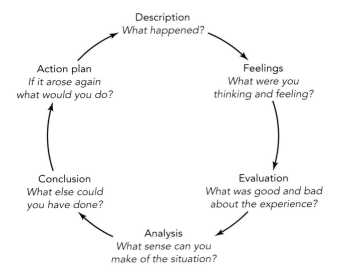

Gibbs' reflective cycle.

Activity

Use Gibbs' six questions to reflect on a situation from your recent experience of supporting a person with a learning disability. Write down your answers. If possible discuss this activity with your line manager or an experienced work colleague.

1. *What happened?*
2. *What were you thinking and feeling?*
3. *What was good and bad about the experience?*
4. *What sense can you make of the situation?*
5. *What else could you have done?*
6. *If it arose again what would you do?*

Thinking point

Reflecting on the support you provide to people every day will help you become more aware of their needs and more person centred in your day-to-day work. Keeping your reflections and looking back on them occasionally will help you to see how much you have developed.

How can I demonstrate that I am a reflective worker?

There a number of different ways to demonstrate that you are a reflective worker. You may need to do this as part of your supervision, for evidence towards a qualification or to show your manager or other colleagues that you are developing in your role.

You can demonstrate your skills as a reflective worker by:

- keeping a learning log or journal of your reflections;

- discussing your ideas with your line manager at your next supervision, using the six questions above as the basis of your discussion;

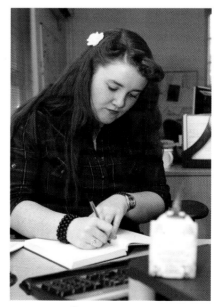

Being a reflective worker – keeping a learning log.

- discussing your ideas and reflections at your next team meeting or with a family carer, get feedback on your ideas to help you become a reflective worker;

- asking a colleague of a person with a learning disability or family carer to provide a witness statement setting out what you have done and how it has changed your practice.

Key points from this chapter

- Think about your own values and attitudes, and talk to others about theirs.

- Listen to the person you are supporting and learn more about their strengths, dreams and needs.

- Read the Code of Practice and other documents that set out the standards you need to work to.

- Listen carefully to any compliments or complaints and take action when it's needed.

- Reflective practice is an important way to learn how to provide good support. It is important because it helps you to understand your own values and attitudes and question what you do.

Chapter 3

Evaluating your performance

> How do I know if I am working in a really person-centred way? Am I doing a good job or could I be doing things differently or better? It would be good to know, and then I could do something about it if I needed to.
>
> *Eleesha, personal assistant to Krista*

Introduction

Sometimes it's difficult to know if you are doing a good job or whether you have improved in an area you once found difficult. Having feedback from others is important, as is being able to evaluate your own performance.

In social care work it is important to have a certain level of communication and number skills so that you can provide good support and keep people safe.

Learning outcomes

This chapter looks at:

- assessing your knowledge, skills and performance against standards;
- using feedback to improve your performance;
- understanding the literacy, numeracy and communication skills needed for your role;
- ways to assess your literacy, numeracy and communication skills.

> **This chapter covers:**
>
> Common Induction Standards – Standard 2 – Personal development: Learning Outcomes 2.2, 3.1 and 3.2
>
> Level 2 SHC 22 – Introduction to personal development: Learning Outcome 2.3
>
> Level 3 SHC 32 – Engage in personal development: Learning Outcome 3.1

Assess my knowledge, skills and performance against standards

As a worker supporting people with a learning disability you will be required to assess your own knowledge, skills and performance in a number of situations. This could include: on completion of your induction or probation period; when you are doing a qualification; at your annual appraisal or when you are applying for a promotion or new job. Assessing your knowledge, skills and performance will also help you as you prepare your personal development plan, looking forward to what more you need to learn to do a good job.

Activity

Answer the three questions below as a way of assessing your competence against different standards.

1. *Are you able to describe the duties and responsibilities of your work role?*

    (a) Yes, I can fully describe my duties and responsibilities.

    (b) I can partly describe my duties and responsibilities.

    (c) I cannot describe my duties and responsibilities yet.

2. *Can you demonstrate your ability to reflect on practice?*

    (a) Yes, I could demonstrate this in several different ways, e.g. from my reflective journal, and from my manager's notes from supervision.

    (b) I can demonstrate this only in one way at the moment; I am working on being more reflective and being able to show what I do.

    (c) No, I can't demonstrate this yet; I have only just learnt about reflective practice and I need to work on this.

3. *As a social care worker are you able to explain how you protect the rights and promote the interests of service users and carers by respecting and maintaining their dignity and privacy? (taken from the GSCC Code of Practice.)*

   (a) *Yes, I am able to provide plenty of evidence that I respect people's dignity and privacy, for example in the way I provide personal care and keep people's personal files safe.*

   (b) *Maybe I could give one or two examples of this, such as last week I didn't give out personal information over the phone about a person I support.*

   (c) *I don't think I can explain how I do this yet; I have only been in my job a few weeks and am still learning about how I would meet these standards.*

Assessing your own performance, knowledge and skills is also important when you are asked to provide support for a new person that you haven't worked with before. Their person centred plan or support plan should tell you what you will be doing with them and the type of support they need. You will need to think through whether you are competent to provide that support. Do you have the right knowledge, skills and attitudes? By breaking down the different parts of a support plan or an externally set standard as the three questions have been above, you will find this fairly easy to do. Another way to assess your competence is to ask other people that you trust to give you feedback on your work.

Using feedback to improve your performance

Getting feedback from the people you support, members of their family, your manager and others will help you to improve the way you work. If you work for an organisation that is inspected, they will receive feedback on their performance from the inspector's report as well as from customer surveys, comments and complaints

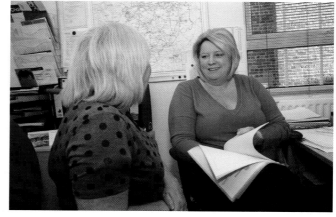

Giving and receiving feedback is one way to assess your performance.

and from any self-assessment they may carry out. Feedback is as important for the organisation as it is for the individual worker. It helps to improve the day-to-day support for people with a learning disability. It is a tool for improvement and development.

You should be open to receiving feedback. Sometimes it can be challenging and difficult to take, particularly if it is given in a negative manner. Some people find it hard to accept feedback even when it is given in a supportive and constructive manner, so you might find it helpful to prepare for feedback on your performance.

In supervision or other more formal situations where you will receive feedback on your work, prepare yourself by:

- asking for feedback both on what you are doing well and on the areas you need to develop;
- having an attitude that all feedback is valuable and useful and can help you develop;
- asking for further information on how you could develop and improve;
- trying not to be defensive – accept what is said, and thank the person for being honest with you – if you are able to, ask for their ideas about how you might improve your performance.

Once you have feedback on your performance you can use this valuable information to improve how you work. You can do this by:

- reflecting on the information using the Gibbs six stage reflection cycle described in Chapter 2;
- identifying any learning needs you might have and adding them to your development plan;
- discussing the feedback with your manager and together keeping your personal development plan up to date.

Why are literacy, numeracy and communication skills important in support work?

Good communication is central to providing good support. So is being able to understand and use information from different people and places. For workers supporting people with a learning disability this means having good language and number skills so that you can provide effective and safe care.

Reading (literacy) and number (numeracy) skills are also important in many jobs supporting people with a learning disability. Do you do any of the following activities during your day-to-day support of a person with a learning disability?

- Read a support plan or person centred plan so you know what support you should be providing.

- Complete an entry in a diary or handover report and read earlier entries from colleagues.

- Read a policy or procedure so you know what to do in a certain situation.

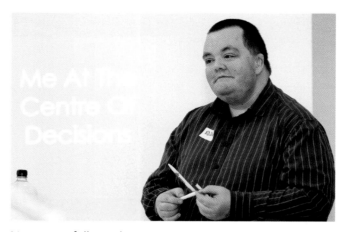
Listen carefully to the person you support.

- Read and complete a medication chart.

- Read and explain a letter for someone.

- Support a person to write a shopping list or menu, following a recipe or cooking instructions.

- Complete a timesheet.

- Listen carefully to a person you support, act on what they say and pass on information accurately and as appropriate to others.

- Discuss a particular issue with workers from another organisation.

- Support a person with their bills and to manage their money within a budget.

- Complete a report.

If your answer to any of these questions is yes, but you struggle with them, then you may need some support with your literacy, numeracy or communication skills. Many people find it difficult to tell others that they might need help with numeracy and literacy skills. However, if you want to do a good job supporting people with a learning disability then you may need to address these issues.

There can be serious consequences for the people that you support if you are not confident with your functional skills (reading, maths and communication). For example:

- the care plan is not followed and the person is put at risk;

- medication is wrongly administered;

- reports and handover documents are not written or are not clear and as a result poor care is provided;
- the person's accounts or budget are not filled in and money is not properly accounted for.

For you as a worker you may not get the correct wages if you find it difficult to fill in your timesheet, and you may find trying to cover up for your lack of skills very stressful. You don't get to appointments on time because you find it hard to find your way or you avoid talking to others because you lack the confidence to pass on information or discuss an important issue. Some of these difficulties can be avoided or addressed if you understand your literacy, numeracy and communication skills and are willing to seek help to develop your skills if you need to. The first step is to assess your skills.

Thinking point

How important do you think good communication skills are to providing support to people with a learning disability? Many jobs also require skills in reading, writing and number. Workers who have difficulty with these skills can get support to develop in their job.

Assessing your literacy, numeracy and communication skills

You can assess your literacy, numeracy and communication skills in a number of different ways.

1. Your employer can do this with you using many of the resources on the Care Skillsbase website at www.scie-careskillsbase.org.uk. The website has lots of checklists that are written specifically for people working in health and social care and so will be relevant to the skills needed in your job.

2. If you are taking a course at a local college or are doing an apprenticeship then you may well have been asked to undertake a functional skills test. This will help staff identify the right support for you.

3. You can also assess your own skills on a number of websites such as www.move-on.org.uk. Also on this website they provide information on the nearest test centre to you so you could go to one for a formal assessment of your literacy, numeracy and IT skills.

If you want to improve your skills then there a number of different things you can do:

- You could talk to your manager and ask for support in your workplace. Your employer should be able to access funding to help them provide this learning for you.

- You could use the Move On website to find your local centre www.move-on.org.uk

- You could ask at your local college or adult education centre about literacy, numeracy and IT assessment and classes.

- Many classes are free or have a small fee and are at different times of the day and evening so that they are suitable for people working different hours.

Key points from this chapter

- Being able to honestly assess your own performance, knowledge and skills against external standards will help you to develop in your role supporting people with a learning disability. You can use self-evaluation and feedback from others to help you.

- Constructive feedback on your performance will help you develop as a worker. You can use feedback to plan your future learning and development.

- Assessing your literacy, numeracy and communication skills will help you know if you need support to develop in this area. Getting help is easy; speak to your manager about this.

References and where to go for more information

References

Skills for Care (2009) *Skills for life – a practical guide for social care employers.* Downloadable from www.skillsforcare.org.uk

Websites

Care Skillsbase www.scie-careskillsbase.org.uk for information for social care employers on assessing literacy and numeracy skills

Move On www.move-on.org.uk for information and mini-tests on literacy and numeracy

Chapter 4

Agreeing your personal development plan and developing your knowledge and skills

I want to do a good job supporting Farooq and Naseer and I needed to learn a lot when I started work. I have learnt so much from Farooq and Naseer and also from their families who have lots of involvement in their lives. After my induction and probation period my manager got me to do a personal development plan and over the last 11 months I have been on a course about person centred working and one on epilepsy support. Jack my colleague has taught me how to support Naseer when he goes for his regular checkups at the doctors. I am now starting to do the diploma in health and social care at the local college. I will be reviewing my plan soon, looking at what I have learnt and looking at what I need to find out over the next year.

Amir, support worker

Introduction

The quality of the support an organisation provides to a person with a learning disability is very closely linked with the quality of the staff it employs. Good organisations understand that the personal development of all of its workers is vital to the provision of a quality service. While your organisation will have put in place systems such as those described below to enable its staff to develop knowledge and skills, it's also up to you to take responsibility for your own learning.

Personal development is equally important for personal assistants (PAs) employed directly by a person with a learning disability or their family carers. A PA needs to work with their employer to identify their learning and development needs and how these will be met.

When you begin your job working with people with learning disabilities you will have induction training. The length of the training and how it is delivered will vary between employers. However, this should be just the start of your personal development as a learning disability worker. You will probably have been employed because you demonstrated that you had the right values and attitudes or because of the knowledge and skills you already have. Your employer may also have seen the potential you have as an individual to gain new skills and knowledge and develop both in your present role and in future roles within the organisation. It is your responsibility to make the most of the opportunities that are presented to gain new skills and knowledge through the process of continuous professional development.

Learning outcomes

This chapter looks at:

- producing a personal development plan;
- sources of support for your learning and development;
- developing and recording progress in your personal development plan;
- reviewing and updating your personal development plan;
- demonstrating the effectiveness of a learning activity;
- using feedback to develop your knowledge and skills.

This chapter covers:

Common Induction Standards – Standard 2 – Personal development: Learning Outcomes 4 and 5

Level 2 SHC 22 – Introduction to personal development: Learning Outcomes 3 and 4

Level 3 SHC 32 – Engage in personal development: Learning Outcomes 4 and 5

Producing a personal development plan

A personal development plan is a record of your learning and development needs that is produced with your employer. The aim of the plan is to help you to develop in your role as a learning disability worker and to help your organisation provide excellent support. In some organisations such a plan might be called a professional development plan or an individual training plan but the overall aim is the same: to identify and plan a person's learning activities.

The personal development process

While documentation varies between organisations, there are generally four stages to the personal development process.

Stage 1 – Identifying your development needs This is the most difficult stage for some people. You will be asked to examine what you feel you are good at and what you need to improve. For example, 'I am good at supporting Susie with the housework and laundry on the days she is at home, but recently when she refused to tidy and clean her room I didn't know what to do for the best.'

Stage 2 – Action planning You need to set targets for building on your strengths and working on areas that you need to improve. For example, 'I need to be able to support Greg better with choice and decision making and understand his likes and dislikes better.'

Stage 3 – Implementing the plan Here you can identify what you need to do in order to meet your targets. You should monitor this regularly. In some organisations you will be asked to identify in your plan any courses you wish to attend or qualifications you wish to achieve. This is because your employer would like you to provide evidence of your commitment to achieving the qualification before they pay for the course, or claim funding. For example, 'When I have finished my induction I need to go on the course on person centred working. I could also read books in the library on supporting choice.'

Stage 4 – Reviewing the plan Reviewing is an important part of the personal development planning process. If it is to be effective, the plan should be a working document which you should look at regularly to keep track of how things are going, and assess whether the targets you set are still relevant and realistic. Your review forms the basis for your next personal development plan. For example, 'I have put into practice some of the lessons I learnt on the course and now understand what Greg likes and dislikes. This has helped me to support him better with day-to-day choices.'

Involving people with learning disabilities and family carers in your personal development plan

The first stage of the process can often be the hardest. Sometimes it's easier to think of our weaknesses than our strengths, and it can be difficult to ask for and hear other people's opinions of how well we do our job. However, it's important to do this so we get a clear picture of our strengths and areas for development.

Your line manager may well help you to do this as part of the process, but it's also

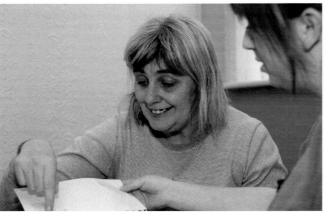

If you feel able to involve the people you support in your personal development plan, not only are you treating them with respect, but you will get a clear picture of how you are seen by the people who are central to your role.

a good idea to find out from the people you support how they see you. If they can communicate verbally, you could ask them to help you think about things you do well, or how you could do some things better. If the person doesn't communicate verbally, you'll be able to tell how they feel about the way you support them by observing them. If you feel able to involve the people you support and their family carer in your personal development plan, not only are you treating them with respect, but you will get a clear picture of how you are seen by the people who are central to your role.

Thinking point

If your friends or family say something good about you, how do you feel? How well do you respond to constructive criticism?

When involving people with learning disabilities and family carers in discussing the support you provide and your development plan, you need to be aware of the power issues involved. Some people may find it easier to talk to someone else about these issues, not to you. If they prefer to be involved in this way you should respect their decision.

The documents each organisation uses to record personal development plans can vary. You will find a useful example in the Skills for Care book *Keeping up the good work – A practical guide to implementing continuing professional development in the adult social care workforce* if you are unfamiliar with the type of paperwork to use.

Sources of support for your learning and development

As a new worker or volunteer you are not expected to know everything about your role or the organisation you work for all at once. One of the exciting things about being a learning disability worker is that you will meet new situations and experiences all the time. Don't be afraid to seek advice, information and support when you need it. This could be from seven main sources.

- The people you support are in the best position to comment on the kind of support they need, and they may have lots of information and knowledge about other things, such as their own disability, wider issues in the learning disability community, events or activities in the local community that they would like to access.

- Family carers usually have a wealth of information about the person you are supporting and most are very willing to share information with new support workers.

- Colleagues can provide emotional support in difficult situations and a wealth of experience and advice. Sharing individually and in team meetings can be helpful for workers.

- Managers can provide information and advice about policies and procedures in your organisation, your job description and role and about your work setting. Don't be afraid to seek support from your manager in difficult situations. Managers or senior workers can mentor new staff in the workplace, teaching them new skills and giving them time to reflect on their work.

- Written information such as policies and procedures, and the aims and values of your organisation, can be found in the staff handbook which you may have received during your induction. Make sure you are familiar with this document and know where to find the information you may need in the future. Your organisation may also hold these documents on its intranet. If you need general information on wider learning disability issues you may find it in your organisation's library. Alternatively, you can contact organisations such as BILD which provide information for new workers.

- Websites and e-learning materials are a source of information for people who have access to a computer either through work, at home or through their local library. A vast amount of information is available on the internet, but you need to be careful that it is accurate and current. One way of doing this is to make sure that the site you get information from is trustworthy. Some reputable websites are listed at the end of this chapter.

- Training events and courses have traditionally been the way that many organisations provide learning for their staff. They are a structured way to learn new skills and knowledge.

Types of learning and development

During your induction as a new worker you are likely to be given information about how the organisation trains and develops its staff. There may be a training manager who is responsible for all training in the organisation, and the organisation may employ trainers who will deliver some or all of the training. The service might employ outside organisations with specialist expertise to deliver some of the training, for example first aid, food hygiene or moving and handling.

However, gaining knowledge and learning new skills isn't just about attending as many training courses and taking as many qualifications as you can, there are many other ways in which this can happen. The people you support, your colleagues and family carers are often excellent sources of information for new workers and you should always be open to asking others if there is something you are unsure about.

Here are some examples of how one support worker gained new knowledge and skills during one week in his new role.

Learning and development examples from Kevin, who supports Louis, Marianne and Terry

Situation/activity	What I learned so I could do a good job in this situation
Louis was going to the dentist and felt worried about having a filling	I asked Louis and his Dad about how to support him well I looked at Louis' support plan to carefully reread the information on supporting him to go to the dentist I talked to Kay, my manager and Louis' key worker, to check what to do
Marianne said her work experience at the supermarket will turn into a paid job soon, but she was not sure about her benefits and all her expenses	Marianne has support at work from GOJOBS, a supported employment agency. I asked them for information on benefits when you start work I talked to Marianne about getting independent expert advice and we made an appointment at the Citizens Advice Bureau. She asked me to go with her and I took notes I asked Kay about how she has supported other people with doing a budget and then I worked through this with Marianne after we got the benefits advice

Terry said the local youths have started calling him names again and he is worried about going out of the house in the evening and at weekends

A few months ago I went on a course about hate crime run by the local self-advocacy group and the police. I got out my notes and read them through carefully

I looked on the internet for accessible information on hate crime to share with Terry

I talked through how I should support Terry with my line manager

Activity

Think about your work supporting people with a learning disability over the last two weeks. Note down some of the things you have learned and the situation you learned them in. What was your best learning experience? Discuss what you have written with your line manager in your next supervision session.

We are all different and people learn in different ways. Finding out about your learning style can help you to learn more effectively. There are a number of theories about learning. One identifies four different learning styles. It says that some people are activist and learn best by doing a task. Pragmatists like to focus on an idea and how it might work in practice. People who like to understand a theory first and enjoy seeing the big picture before considering the application of an idea are called theorists. And finally reflectors prefer to stand back and think about an idea or experience before taking action. There are lots of ways to find out what type of learner you are. There are quizzes in books and on the internet. When you are planning your own learning and development, knowing how you like to learn can help you to plan effective learning that best suits your needs.

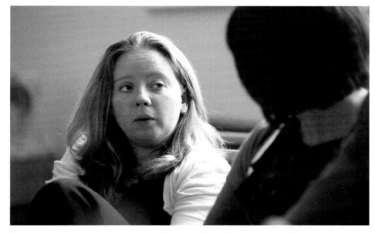

You can gain new knowledge and skills informally from your colleagues and the people you support.

Gaining new knowledge and skills can take place formally in training sessions and informally as you learn from people with learning disabilities, their relatives, your colleagues and managers.

Developing and recording a personal development plan

We make plans every day about what we need to do and how we are going to go about it. We may write some of these down. A personal development plan is a written plan in which you identify the knowledge and skills you need to equip you to provide high quality support and to develop your career. Personal development is important for learning disability workers in small and large organisations as well as those who are directly employed by the person they support. In social care it is important that both new and experienced workers have a personal development plan, because when you are new you need to learn a lot. As a more experienced worker you need to learn new skills because the needs of the people you support might change, and the laws, standards and policies and procedure in your organisation can change. You are also able to take on new roles and responsibilities in the future because social care is changing all the time and you need to be flexible and respond to changing needs.

As a worker supporting a person with learning disabilities this means that when you start in social care work you will undergo an induction and then overtime undertake further learning and development to:

- give you the knowledge and skills so that you can provide high quality support;
- enable your employer to ensure that you are safe and capable to carry out your job;
- prepare you for new responsibilities;
- help you progress in your career.

Once you have identified your learning needs, then you need to devise an action plan to achieve them. You are not expected to do this on your own. Most organisations have a procedure for personal development planning and a document which you should complete with the help of your line manager.

SAMPLE personal development form

Name – Jackie Jones

Place of work – from the south Bristol office supporting people in their own home and the community

Date completed – January 2011

Date to be reviewed – April 2011

What I want or need to learn over the next 12 months.

Learning needed	Date to be completed	How to achieve the learning	How I put the learning into practice
I want to learn more about community connecting to support Elsie and Alice to join in activities at the community centre	end of April 2011	Go on the half day course at head office in March Read the book that Eva recommended Talk to colleagues about their experiences and what they would pass on as good practice	
Urgently need to learn how to support Mickey with his new hearing aid	next two weeks	Read through with Mickey the information he got from the hearing aid centre and talk with him about what has worked Look for advice for new hearing aid users on the internet Talk to Ryan (a manager who is a learning disability nurse) for more information on how deafness can affect people with a learning disability	

Learning needed	Date to be completed	How to achieve the learning	How I put the learning into practice
I still want to explore applying for a nursing course in a few years so want to take the level 3 diploma in the next 18 months	aim to start course within 6 months	Talk to the training manager about my options Get prospectuses from two local colleges Find out about funding Look on the internet to find out more about the diploma options	

Reviewing and updating your personal development plan

Your personal development plan should be a living document, not something you fill in and then put in your file for six months. At your supervisions you should look at your personal development plan with your line manager. There should also be regular points during the year, maybe every three or four months, when at your supervision you formally review your progress. Getting into the habit of making notes about what you have learnt and how you have put the idea or skill into practice will definitely help you to develop as a reflective practitioner.

Demonstrate the effectiveness of a learning activity

Of course learning for its own sake is important, but when you are undertaking learning for your job, your employer and the people you support will want to know whether the learning you have undertaken has actually been useful and that you are competent. There are a number of different ways that you can demonstrate the effectiveness of a learning activity.

- You are able to safely show that you can do a task that you couldn't do before, e.g. use a fire extinguisher, use a hoist, administer medication.
- You are able to use your knowledge to improve the way you support a person, e.g. a course on good communication has enabled you to be an active listener and you now pay much more attention to the body language and facial expression of the people you support.
- You keep a learning log to reflect on your learning.
- Changing the way you work – for example, after going on a course about partnership working with family carers you show more respect for the family carers you meet and show that you value their experience and knowledge.

Key points from this chapter

- A personal development plan should be a living document. It is important that you keep it up to date and review it regularly with your supervisor.

References and where to go for more information
References

Skills for Care (2010) *Keeping up the good work – a practical guide to implementing continuing professional development in the adult social care workforce.* Downloadable from www.skillsforcare.org.uk

Websites

Action for Advocacy www.actionforadvocacy.org.uk

British Institute of Learning Disabilities: www.bild.org.uk

Circles Network www.circlesnetwork.org.uk

Communication Matters www.communicationmatters.org.uk

Department of Health www.dh.gov.uk

Foundation for People with Learning Disabilities: www.learningdisabilities.org.uk

Makaton www.makaton.org

Mencap www.mencap.org.uk

Signalong www.signalong.org.uk

Glossary

Aims a general statement of what an organisation hopes to achieve

Code of practice a UK document for social care workers setting out the standards they should be working to

Continuous professional development or CPD is learning that you undertake after your induction that will help you develop in your role or that will advance your career

Confidentiality things that need to be kept private

Direct payments a way for people to organise their own social care support by receiving funding direct from their council following an assessment of their needs

Family carer a relative of a person with learning disabilities who has an interest in their wellbeing

General Social Care Council the organisation that regulates the social care workforce in England and sets the standards of care through the Codes of Practice

Induction a period of learning, shortly after starting a new job or volunteering placement, about how to provide good support to people with learning disabilities

Job description a document that gives detailed information about your work, what you will be doing, who you are responsible to, etc.

Person centred approach a way of working every day with people with learning disabilities that puts the person and their dreams at the centre of everything you do

Personal development plan a plan completed by a worker with their manager to record their future learning and development needs

Policy a statement or plan of action that clearly sets out an organisation's position or approach on a particular issue and tells staff what should be done in the circumstances

Procedure a set of instructions which sets out in detail how a policy should be implemented and what staff should do in response to a specific situation

Reflection careful consideration of ideas and issues

Rights legal protection that protects from harm, sets out what people can say and do and guarantees the right to a fair trial and other basic entitlements, such as the right to respect, equality, etc.

Service the provision of social care support for a person that could be in their own home, their local community, a residential home or similar place

Support plan a detailed plan of a person's support needs that support workers should use to inform their day-to-day support for that individual

Index

Added to a page number 'g' denotes glossary.